Flex Nutrition

Supplements to Elevate your Fitness Game

Table of Contents

Chapter 1. Introduction

Discover the undeniable power of Flex Nutrition in our latest Special Report: "Flex Nutrition: Supplements to Elevate your Fitness Game". Get ready to elevate your fitness journey to new heights in a world of natural supplements, precise meal plans, and groundbreaking insights – all tailored to your unique body needs. Whether you're a fitness enthusiast or just starting your journey, this report is designed for every stride and pace. Equal parts informative and motivating, this Special Report will make you eager to lace up your running shoes, prepare that power smoothie, and seize your fitness destiny – one well-nourished step at a time. So, are you ready to start your adventure towards ultimate fitness? This Special Report is your ticket to a healthier, stronger, and more energetic you. Get your copy today; let the games begin!

Chapter 2. Understanding Supplements: The Foundations and Basics

With the right balance of diet and exercise, supplements can provide the necessary kick to elevate your fitness journey. However, understanding these products is crucial before incorporating them into your routine.

2.1. The Role of Supplements in Fitness

Dietary supplements are substances you might use to add nutrients to your diet or to lower your risk of health problems. They could include vitamins, minerals, amino acids, herbs, or enzymes packed in pills, capsules, powders, or liquids.

Even though supplements are often viewed in the context of athletic enhancement, their fundamental role is health optimization. Their primary purpose is to complement your diet and make up for any nutrients that might be lacking in your usual foods. They can also help boost specific bodily functions or conditions based on their constituents.

However, supplements are not designed to replace entire food groups or a balanced diet. They are meant to bridge nutritional gaps. Committing to a healthy, balanced diet is a must, irrespective of whether you're consuming supplements or not.

2.2. Understanding the Types of Supplements

The world of supplements can be divided into several types, primarily based on their ingredients and the purpose they serve.

- **Protein Supplements:** These are the most popular in the fitness industry. They aid in muscle recovery, growth, and repair post-workout. Unsurprisingly, they are particularly favored by strength and endurance athletes.

- **Creatine Supplements:** Known for enhancing physical performance and aiding muscle gain.

- **Vitamin and Mineral Supplements:** These make up for potential deficiencies in our diet. For example, Vitamin D is commonly taken in areas with low sun exposure.

- **Branched-Chain Amino Acid (BCAA) Supplements:** Useful in muscle recovery and reducing muscle soreness.

- **Pre-Workout Supplements:** As the name suggests, these are taken prior to a workout to enhance performance and energy levels.

- **Post-Workout Supplements:** Taken after a workout, they help recover lost nutrients and mend damaged muscles.

While choosing a supplement, it's crucial to do your research. Not all supplements are created equal, and each has a unique impact based on the ingredients and their efficacy.

2.3. The Impact of Overuse and Misuse

Equally important is understanding the dangers of supplement misuse. The key to getting the most benefits from your supplements lies in using them at the right dosage and timing. Overuse or misuse can lead to several unwanted health problems.

For example, excessive consumption of protein powder can have harmful effects on your kidneys and liver. Therefore, it's important to adhere to the dosage recommended by health professionals or the manufacturer.

Also, remember that supplements are just that – supplementary to your diet. Over-reliance can lead to imbalances in your nutrient intake, which can do more harm than good in the long run.

2.4. Knowing the Importance of Natural Food

While supplements work great, including nutrient-rich foods in your diet is vital. Supplements are meant to supplement the diet, not replace meals. They should never become the primary source of your nutrients. Fruits, vegetables, whole grains, lean meat, dairy, and healthy fats offer complete nutrition, which cannot be replicated by a supplement.

Therefore, one should view supplements as an add-on rather than an alternative to their diet. They help fill dietary gaps and meet increased dietary demands due to exercise, stress, and other factors, but achieving most of your nutrients from a balanced diet is essential.

2.5. Final Thoughts

Supplements can be a substantial booster for your fitness goals when used correctly, but their use should be informed and intentional. Always remember to consult a physician or a certified fitness/nutrition expert before starting a new supplement regimen.

Remember, every supplement won't work the same way for everyone. Everybody is unique, and so are their nutrient requirements. Therefore, understanding and identifying the correct type, amount, and application of supplements is vital for optimum fitness results.

Above all, promoting regular exercise, a balanced diet, and healthy lifestyle habits should always be the priority. The power of proper nutrition combined with intelligent supplementation can lead to enhanced performance, better recovery, and overall improved health.

Chapter 3. Decoding Nutritional Labels: Your Guide to Smart Supplement Selection

What we consume, especially when it comes to supplements, can play a pivotal role in our fitness journey. This is where the significance of understanding nutritional labels comes in. They serve as a roadmap to guide us in making smart supplement selections.

3.1. Understanding Basic Nutritional Terminologies

Before diving into the world of nutritional labels, let's understand a few basic terminologies that you'll encounter.

- **Calories:** The energy content in food is calculated in units of calories. We need a specific number of calories to function, and excess calories result in weight gain.

- **Macronutrients:** These are the nutrients our bodies need in large amounts: carbohydrates, proteins, and fats.

- **Micronutrients:** These are nutrients needed in smaller quantities like vitamins and minerals.

- **Dietary Fiber:** This is a type of carbohydrate that the body can't fully digest. It aids in digestion and can help prevent heart disease, diabetes, weight gain, and certain types of cancer.

3.2. Decoding the Serving Size

Nutritional labels start with the serving size, which is a standardized amount that helps you compare similar foods and supplements. It isn't a recommendation of how much you should eat or drink. The serving size will dictate the amount of calories and nutrients on the label. So, a supplement may contain 2 servings, and when you consume the whole thing, you're actually getting double the calories and nutrients.

3.3. Analyzing Caloric Content

Next in line on the nutritional label is the number of calories per serving. If you're trying to gain, lose, or maintain weight, paying attention to the caloric content of supplements is crucial. Remember, not all calories are created equal. 100 calories from a candy bar impacts your body differently than 100 calories from a protein bar. Your goal should be to opt for supplements rich in nutritious calories.

3.4. Making Sense of Macronutrients

Macronutrients - carbohydrates, proteins, and fats - contribute to the calorie content of the product. Understanding how to read macronutrients on the label can help you choose the right supplement depending on your dietary needs.

- **Carbohydrates:** There are three types: sugars, starches, and fiber. While sugars are simple carbs and provide quick energy, starches and fiber are complex carbs and are digested more slowly, providing a sustained energy source.

- **Proteins:** The building block of muscles; essential if you're looking to build strength and muscle mass. A high protein content in your supplement is desirable if you're a bodybuilder or training intensively.

- **Fats:** While fats are high in calories, they're essential for many body functions. Healthy fats such as omega-3 fatty acids support heart health and can be beneficial in a fitness regime.

3.5. Evaluating Micronutrients

Even though required in lesser quantities, micronutrients are crucial for overall health and fitness. The inclusion of essential minerals and vitamins – the typical micronutrients – in your supplements can significantly boost their nourishing power.

3.6. Deciphering the Ingredients List

The ingredients list provides information about what is included in the supplement. Ingredients are listed in descending order by weight – the first ingredient listed contributes the most to the product, while the last adds the least. In general, shorter lists with recognizable ingredients are preferable.

3.7. The % Daily Value

The % Daily Value (%DV) tells you the percentage of each nutrient in a single serving, in terms of the daily recommended amount. It can help you determine if a product is high or low in a specific nutrient. As a general guide, 5% DV or less is low and 20% DV or more is high.

Understanding how to navigate nutritional labels is an invaluable skill. It can serve as your guiding compass, enabling the creation of a tailored nutritional intake that is in sync with your fitness goals. By mastering this skill, you can leverage the transformative power of nutrition to fuel your fitness quest strategically and sustainably. Be patient with yourself as you practice this new nutritional literacy; it is sure to pay off in terms of maximized workout results and optimized overall health.

Chapter 4. Protein Powders: Building Blocks of Muscle Growth

We all know that proteins play a vital role in our bodies' functions. They aid in repairing body cells, making new ones, and contributing to our overall muscle growth. Protein powders are an excellent means to ensure you're getting the right amount of protein your body needs to fuel your muscle growth and recovery, especially if you're leading an active lifestyle.

4.1. Types of Protein Powders

There are various types of protein powders available on market. Each type has its benefits and uses, depending on individual's needs and lifestyle.

1. **Whey**: The most common type, whey protein, is a water-soluble milk protein. It's complete, which means it includes all 9 essential amino acids. It's also high in the amino acid leucine, crucial for muscle protein synthesis.

2. **Casein**: This type of protein is also derived from milk. It's digested and absorbed more slowly compared to whey, offering a steady stream of amino acid release to fuel your muscles.

3. **Soy**: For those allergic to dairy or practicing a vegan lifestyle, soy is the best alternative. It's a complete plant-based protein and rich in antioxidants.

4. **Pea**: Pea protein has gained popularity for being a plant-based alternative comparable to whey in effectiveness. It's also hypoallergenic and high in BCAAs, making it a popular choice among vegans and those with specific dietary restrictions.

5. **Rice**: Although not a complete protein, it's hypoallergenic and easy to digest. Often, you'll see rice protein combined with pea protein to form a complete amino acid profile.

6. **Hemp**: This is also a plant-based protein full of omega-3 and omega-6 fatty acids. It's easily digestible but doesn't provide as high a protein content per serving as others.

4.2. Selecting the Right Protein Powder

The ingredients listing and nutritional label are your best friends when it comes to selecting the ideal protein powder. Look for a product with a high protein count (usually ranging between 20 to 30 grams per serving) and low sugar content.

It's also essential to pay attention to any additional ingredients that might align with your wellness goals. Some powders may contain added BCAAs, greens, or probiotics to further enhance your muscle growth and overall health.

One significant factor to consider is potential allergies or dietary restrictions. Be mindful of any intolerances you may have, and choose a protein powder that aligns with your dietary needs.

4.3. Incorporating Protein Powder into Your Diet

There's an array of ways you can incorporate protein powders into your diet. Some prefer the classic route — mixing it with water or milk for a post-workout shake. But you can also sprinkle protein powder on your smoothie, yogurt, or morning bowl of oatmeal. Baking protein powder into muffins or pancake batter is another delicious way to consume it.

Remember, the key is consistency. It's not just about taking protein powder right after every workout but incorporating it into your daily diet to ensure a steady supply of protein for muscle growth and repair.

4.4. Understanding Your Protein Needs

Your protein needs will be correlated with your body weight, the intensity of your physical activity, and your muscle building goals. To calculate your protein requirement, a general rule of thumb is 1.2-2.0 grams of protein per kilogram of body weight.

Keep in mind, these are general recommendations and can vary drastically depending upon individual needs. A dietitian can provide guidance tailored to your unique body needs and help you understand your protein needs better.

4.5. Potential Side Effects and Precautions

Though protein powders are relatively safe for most people, taking too much can lead to adverse effects. Over-consumption of protein can lead to digestive problems like bloating, gas, and in severe cases, damage to kidneys.

It's essential to balance your protein intake with other macronutrients. A well-rounded diet is key to achieving optimal muscle growth and general health. Always remember, supplements like protein powders should supplement your diet, not replace whole foods.

In Conclusion, protein powders offer a convenient, versatile, and efficient way to increase your protein intake and promote muscle growth. They're a reliable ally on your fitness journey; just remember to choose wisely and consume responsibly to capitalize on their benefits and avoid potential downsides. This way, you'll be well on your way to breaking new records, reaching your fitness goals, and leading a healthier, more nourishing lifestyle. Remember, your journey to ultimate fitness is a marathon, not a sprint, and every well-nourished step is a stride towards victory.

Do this right, and you may soon find yourself eager to lace up those running shoes or prepare that power smoothie — all with the help of the right protein powder by your side. Let's take on the road to ultimate fitness, well-nourished and stronger than ever. Together, we lift.

Chapter 5. Pre-Workout Supplements: Unleash the Full Potential of your Workouts

Pre-workout supplements are designed to boost your performance, energy, and focus, enabling you to get the most out of each training session. Scientific advances and studies in the field of sports nutrition have led to innovative, natural mixtures, which can support the body before, during, and after a workout. In this chapter, we will delve into the benefits of different supplements, debunk common misconceptions, and guide you on how to use them to your advantage.

5.1. Understanding Pre-Workout Supplements

Before we dive into the various options on the market, it is important to understand what pre-workout supplements are, and how they can aid in your training regimen. A pre-workout supplement is usually a powdered substance that you mix with water and consume before exercise. They are designed to increase your energy, endurance, and focus during a workout. These products achieve their effects through a blend of different ingredients, such as caffeine, BCAAs (branch chain amino acids), creatine, beta-alanine, and citrulline malate, each of which we will break down in the course of this chapter.

5.2. Components of Pre-Workout Supplements

As we have already mentioned, pre-workout supplements are concoctions of various ingredients that are designed to optimize physical performance. Let's take a closer look.

- **Caffeine** – Known for its stimulating effects, caffeine enhances alertness and reduces the perception of effort, which allows for longer and more intense workouts.

- **BCAAs (branch chain amino acids)** – These are essential amino acids: leucine, isoleucine, and valine, which support muscle growth and recovery.

- **Creatine** – This substance is naturally present in muscle cells and plays a critical role in energy production during high-intensity workouts.

- **Beta-Alanine** – An amino acid, beta-alanine helps combat muscle fatigue, allowing for more prolonged, intensive training sessions.

- **Citrulline Malate** – This constituent is used for delayed onset muscle soreness (DOMS) and improving exercise performance, by enhancing the production of nitric oxide, which can improve blood flow.

5.3. Benefits of Pre-Workout Supplements

Pre-workout supplements offer varied benefits, depending on their ingredients. Generally, they can assist in improving workout performance and efficiency, enhancing energy and focus, promoting faster muscle growth and speeding recovery, as well as boosting metabolic rate and fat loss.

5.4. Choosing the Right Pre-Workout Supplement

Not all pre-workout supplements are created equal - each come with a unique blend of ingredients and serves different needs. Your ideal choice will depend on your personal fitness goals, tolerance to caffeine, dietary preferences, and budget. When purchasing a pre-workout supplement, one should consider the following elements:

- **Your Fitness Goals** – If your main goal is to build muscle, a product high in BCAAs and creatine would be beneficial. If your goal is to improve endurance, caffeine and beta-alanine would be ideal.

- **Caffeine Sensitivity** – If you are sensitive to caffeine, consider a stimulant-free product.

- **Dietary Restrictions** – If you're on a special diet, like vegan or gluten-free, make sure the product aligns with your dietary needs.

- **Price** – Always compare the price by serving rather than the total cost of the container to understand the real value.

Always consult with a healthcare provider before starting any new supplement regimen, especially if you have underlying health conditions.

5.5. Potential Side Effects and Misuse

While pre-workout supplements can be beneficial, they can also cause side effects if not used properly. Side effects can include heart palpitations, high blood pressure, sleep disturbances, and kidney damage. Overuse or dependency can also lead to withdrawal symptoms like fatigue, irritability, and depression.

In conclusion, pre-workout supplements are powerful tools that, when used properly, can significantly enhance your workout performance and results. However, it's important to understand that supplements are just one piece of the puzzle. A nutritious diet, consistent workout routine, adequate rest, and hydration are also paramount to achieve your fitness goals. If you decide that a pre-workout supplement is right for you, take the time to find a product that meets your specific needs and follow the recommended dosages to ensure the safest and most effective use. With the right approach, the world of pre-workout supplements can provide a valuable boost towards attaining peak fitness – a peak that is not a destination, but a continually evolving journey.

Chapter 6. Vitamins and Minerals: The Silent Heroes for Recovery and Strength

Your body is a complex biological machine that requires various nutrients to function optimally. Among these nutrients, vitamins and minerals hold a unique and important place. Vitamins and minerals are often seen as the 'silent heroes' of recovery and strength and are absolutely essential for maintaining vital body functions, enhancing your workout potential, and aiding in muscle recovery post-exercise.

6.1. The Essential Role of Vitamins and Minerals

Vitamins and minerals, collectively known as micronutrients, are involved in every aspect of bodily function. They contribute to the production of energy in our cells, regulate metabolism, maintain a healthy immune system, play a critical role in healing and recovery, and help to build resistance to diseases. Their role is silent yet indispensable to the overall health and functionality of the human body.

Despite not providing calories or energy directly, vitamins and minerals enable the body to efficiently use energy from the food we eat - a factor that is of immense importance during and after fitness workouts. They are paramount in converting food into energy and repairing cellular damage, making them vital for recovery and strength.

6.2. Understanding Vitamins

Vitamins are organic compounds that the body needs in small quantities for different functions. They are classified into two categories: fat-soluble (A, D, E, K) and water-soluble (C and all the B vitamins). Each type works differently in the body.

Fat-soluble vitamins are stored primarily in the liver and fatty tissues, and they require fat for the body to effectively absorb them. In contrast, water-soluble vitamins are not stored in the body and must be replenished daily. They assist in releasing energy from food, strengthen the immune system, and produce collagen which is vital in muscle tissue repair.

6.3. Understanding Minerals

Minerals, on the other hand, are inorganic substances which the body requires to carry out various functions, including regulation of the body's hydration status, maintaining healthy bones and teeth, and helping in muscle contraction – a phenomenon exceptionally crucial for athletes or anyone working out.

Key minerals like calcium, magnesium, phosphorus, and potassium, among others, regulate important bodily functions. For example, calcium and magnesium are needed for complementing muscle function, while electrolytes like sodium and potassium balance the fluids in the body and prevent muscle cramps during workouts.

6.4. The Fitness Connection: Vitamins and Exercise

The relationship between vitamins, minerals, and exercise is an intimate one. When you exercise, your body uses up more of these essential nutrients as it gears up to repair and recover. For those engaging in regular or high-intensity exercises, this increased demand can only be met with a well-rounded diet or supplementation.

Notably, the B-vitamins are linked to improving athletic performance due to their role in energy production and red blood cell formation. Vitamin C aids in the growth and repair of tissues, hence accelerating the muscle recovery process. Vitamin D paired with calcium supports bones, reduces inflammation, and regulates immune function – all crucial aspects of recovery and strength in fitness.

6.5. The Fitness Connection: Minerals and Exercise

As with vitamins, minerals are crucial for exercise performance. Iron is crucial due to its role in delivering oxygen to the muscles, thus aiding in endurance exercises. Calcium and Vitamin D are vital for bone health and muscle function. When it comes to hydration, the role of electrolytes (sodium and potassium) cannot be emphasized enough. They balance the fluids in your body, help your muscles to contract, and combat muscle cramping, allowing you to perform at your peak during a workout.

6.6. Post-Workout Recovery: The Role of Vitamins and Minerals

Essential nutrients become particularly important during the recovery phase post-workout. During exercise, the body undergoes stress, leading to muscle tissue damage and inflammation. Vitamins and minerals assist in repairing this damage, limiting inflammation, and creating new blood vessels, thereby facilitating efficient recovery.

Key micronutrients for recovery include Vitamin C (for repairing tissues and limiting prolonged inflammation), Vitamin D (for optimal immune function), and the mineral Zinc (contributing to wound healing and the immune response). A deficiency in these nutrients can hamper recovery and limit progress in your fitness journey.

6.7. Nutrient Timing and Absorption

Understanding the timing of nutrient intake can enhance their absorption, ultimately increasing their utilization and benefit to the body. Consuming vitamins and minerals alongside certain foods can improve absorption, such as fat-soluble vitamins alongside high-quality fats, or Vitamin C with iron-rich foods for better iron absorption.

6.8. Conclusion

Considering the critical role that these micronutrients play in supporting overall health and specifically physical fitness, it's essential to ensure an adequate intake of vitamins and minerals. This intake can come from a balanced diet, fortified foods, and possibly supplementation (if needed and under the guidance of a healthcare provider).

This in-depth understanding of the 'silent heroes' - vitamins and minerals, underscores their importance in fitness and recovery. Paying detailed consideration to your micronutrient intake can equip you with the strength, resilience and vitality needed to elevate your performance and progress in your fitness journey. In the world of fitness where focus is often placed on macronutrients like carbohydrates, proteins, and fats, let's not forget the silent yet powerful micronutrients that are the vitamins and minerals.

Chapter 7. Omega-3 Fatty Acids: Powering Up on Heart Health and Joint Flexibility

Omega-3 fatty acids, also known as n-3 fatty acids, are a group of polyunsaturated fats renowned for their numerous health benefits. Extensive research has shown that the body can reap significant benefits from their inclusion in the diet.

These essential fats come in three key types: alpha-linolenic acid (ALA), eicosapentaenoic acid (EPA), and docosahexaenoic acid (DHA). ALA is mainly found in plants, such as flaxseeds and walnuts, while EPA and DHA are commonly found in seafood, particularly fatty fish.

=== Understanding Omega-3 Fatty Acids

Omega-3 fatty acids are crucial for the body's growth and maintenance, but the human body cannot produce them. That's why they are classified as essential – we need to obtain them from our diet or through quality supplements.

Our bodies utilize these fatty acids in numerous ways, including brain function and cell regeneration, but for fitness enthusiasts, they hold particular significance for heart health and joint flexibility. Omega-3 fatty acids are known to reduce inflammation in the body, aid in muscle recovery, and promote overall cardiovascular health.

=== Optimizing Heart Health with Omega-3 Fatty Acids

Several studies have demonstrated the positive impacts of Omega-3 fatty acids on heart health. Notably, consuming Omega-3-rich fish or supplements has been linked to a lower risk of heart disease and stroke, lessened incidences of blood clotting, and reduced levels of triglyceride – a type of fat found in your blood that, in high amounts, can increase chances of heart disease.

Table 1. Omega-3 and Heart Health

Incorporating Omega-3 fatty acids into your routine, whether through diet or supplementation, could help maintain a healthy heart, particularly if you lead an active lifestyle. Regular physical activity coupled with resistance training can sometimes place excess strain on the heart, but Omega-3 fatty acids can help mitigate this risk by maintaining a strong and healthy cardiovascular system.

=== Boosting Joint Flexibility with Omega-3 Fatty Acids

For fitness enthusiasts, regular joint pain or stiffness can become a burden. Fortunately, Omega-3 fatty acids have been found to aid in reducing joint inflammation, increasing blood flow during exercise, and even decreasing morning stiffness.

Table 2. Omega-3 and Joint Health

Paying attention to joint health is vital for those in strength training or endurance sports. Even regular gym-goers can benefit from the improved flexibility and reduced joint discomfort that Omega-3 fatty acids can provide.

=== Implementing Omega-3 Fatty Acids into Your Routine

So, how can you take advantage of these significant benefits? Omega-3 fatty acids can be obtained naturally through a balanced diet rich in fatty fish like salmon, mackerel, and tuna, as well as plant sources such as walnuts and flaxseeds.

For those adverse to fish or unable to manage a consistently balanced diet, Omega-3 supplements offer a convenient alternative. Quality is paramount when choosing supplements – read labels carefully to ensure you're receiving the EPA and DHA necessary for those functional benefits.

Remember to consult your doctor or a nutritionist before starting any supplementation routine, particularly if you are pregnant, nursing, or dealing with a chronic health condition.

Omega-3 fatty acids are a powerhouse when it comes to fostering our heart health and joint flexibility. By incorporating this essential nutrient into our regular routine, we give our bodies the support to keep up with our fitness goals while bolstering our overall health.

Chapter 8. Demystifying Diet: Complementing Supplements with Right Food Choices

The statement 'You are what you eat' couldn't be more truthful, especially when considering the world of fitness and nutrition. Nutrition is a cardinal point of your fitness journey, serving as the fuel to power your body and mind. In essence, your food choices play an integral role in your overall fitness.

8.1. Understanding Supplements and Natural Food

Fundamentally, dietary supplements are intended to augment your daily intake of nutrients, majorly derived from food. They encompass vitamins, minerals, amino acids, and enzymes, offered in myriad forms such as tablets, powders, capsules, liquids, and gummies. Some popular types are Vitamin D, Calcium, Iron, and multivitamins, among others.

However, supplements should never be a substitute for a varied diet. The rule of thumb is that you obtain a majority of your nutrients from foods and use supplements as a 'top-up' where necessary. Real, natural foods come with a complex mix of vitamins, fiber, and minerals that are often deficient in supplements.

8.2. Nutrient Bioavailability: Why It Matters

An essential concept to grasp is the aspect of nutrient bioavailability, which refers to the proportion of a nutrient absorbed and utilized by the body. This rate has a significant impact on the efficacy of both food and supplements in delivering nutrients to the body.

In whole foods, nutrients are, generally, more bioavailable than in supplements. Combining certain foods also magnifies the bioavailability of nutrients. For instance, consuming vitamin C-rich foods like oranges with iron-rich foods like spinach can increase your body's absorption of iron.

8.3. Food-First Approach to Nutrition

The real magic happens when you master the art of combining the right food choices with supplements. A food-first approach should be at the core of your nutrition strategy, ensuring that you prioritize well-balanced meals before considering supplement intake.

A well-rounded diet incorporates a robust mix of macronutrients - proteins, carbohydrates, and fats, alongside micronutrients such as vitamins and minerals. Proteins are the building blocks, aiding muscle repair, and growth, whereas carbohydrates and fats serve as the primary energy sources. Vitamins and minerals, too, play a range of roles in the body from supporting bone health to improving immune function.

Consideration should also be given to pre-workout and post-workout nutrition. Pre-workout meals filled with protein and complex carbohydrates such as a chicken sandwich can provide a sustained energy release. Simultaneously, post-workout nutrition needs to replenish the used glycogen stores and aid in muscle recovery - this is where a protein shake and a banana could come in handy.

8.4. Identifying the Right Supplements for You

Despite the food-first approach, there are scenarios where supplements come in handy. For instance, in situations where nutrient needs are hard to meet through diet alone, such as in strict vegan diets or certain health conditions. Sportspeople or active persons undertaking intense workouts may also need supplementary support.

The key to efficient supplementation is correct identification of what your body needs. This largely hinges on your diet, age, health status, fitness goals, and intensity of physical activity. Common supplements employed in fitness include protein powders, Branched-Chain Amino Acids (BCAAs), beta-alanine, and creatine. Always remember, supplements should supplement, not substitute a healthy diet.

8.5. Demystifying Common Nutritional Myths

As you embark on this journey of marrying the right food with supplements, you might encounter several myths. Prominent ones include thinking that supplements can offset a poor diet, more protein equals larger muscles, and that overweight people need to take dietary supplements. These are falsehoods. Always ensure that your information is based on scientific facts and research.

Nutrition may seem like an intricate web, and while it's possible to navigate it solo, professional help could ease the journey. Nutritionists, dietitians, and trainers can support and guide you in making informed, personalized diet plans and supplement choices.

In conclusion, harmonizing your diet with the right supplements could be your game-changer in recognizing your fitness goals. A food-first approach, coupled with judicious use of supplements, can elevate your performance, pushing you closer to a healthier, fitter, and more energized you. Start today; go slow, go steady, but above all, stay consistent. After all, Rome wasn't built in a day!

Chapter 9. Smoothies and Shakes: Delicious Recipes for Nutrient-Packed Drinks

In the realm of fitness, nutrition occupies a central, non-negotiable position. Consuming the right balance of macronutrients and micronutrients fuels our bodies for peak physical performance and long-lasting health. In this chapter, we've compiled an assortment of delightful smoothie and shake recipes, each carefully designed to provide an explosion of essential nutrients. These delicious concoctions will not only elevate your energy levels, but are also conveniently quick to prepare, perfect for your bustling lifestyle.

9.1. The Basics of a Nutrient-Rich Shake

Before we jump into specific recipes, let's first understand the foundation of a nutrient-packed shake. Every shake should provide you with a balance of quality protein, fiber-packed carbohydrates, and healthy fats – the three key macronutrients our bodies depend on to function optimally. Furthermore, a worthy shake should also be teeming with essential vitamins and minerals. By tying together these elements, we conjure a beverage that is both nutritious and tasty.

Most smoothie and shake recipes follow a common structure:

1. A source of protein (like a scoop of protein powder).

2. A liquid to blend everything together (milk or a milk alternative, such as almond milk).

3. A medley of fruits and/or vegetables.

4. A source of healthy fats (like a dollop of nut butter or a handful of

chia seeds).

5. A source of carbohydrates (usually complex carbs like oats or quinoa).

Now that we've established the basic principles, let's dive into delicious specifics.

9.2. Rise and Shine Smoothie

Incorporate a splash of vibrant sunshine into your morning routine with this energy-boosting smoothie. This recipe is rich in vitamin C and fiber, vital for a robust immune system and a happy gut.

Ingredient list:

- 1 small orange, peeled and segmented

- 1 small banana, sliced and frozen

- 1/2 cup of reduced-fat Greek yogurt

- 1/4 cup raw oats

- 1/2 cup almond milk

- 1 scoop of vanilla protein powder

- 1 tablespoon chia seeds

Blend all the ingredients together until smooth. Enjoy your nutrient-packed sunrise!

9.3. Green Goddess Shake

Packed with protein and loaded with leafy goodness, this shake is a refreshing way to consume your greens. Its unique blend of superfoods will keep you invigorated all day.

Ingredient list:

- 1 scoop of plant-based protein powder

- 1 cup of fresh spinach

- 1 small banana

- 1/2 avocado

- 1 cup of unsweetened almond milk

- 1 tablespoon flax seeds

- Ice as needed

Blend all together until you have a smooth, velvety shake. Sip on your green dream!

9.4. Post-Workout Power Shake

Working out depletes your muscles and energy reserves which need to be replenished. Here is a quick recipe to help refuel with protein, carbs, and necessary electrolytes.

Ingredient list:

- 1 scoop of chocolate protein powder

- 1 small banana

- 1 tablespoon peanut butter

- 8 ounces of coconut water

- 1/4 teaspoon sea salt

- Ice as necessary

Blend all the ingredients until it's smooth and creamy. This post-workout power shake will help your muscles recover and keep hunger pangs at bay.

9.5. The Antioxidant Boost

Harvest the power of antioxidant-rich berries, chia seeds, and protein powder to boost your immunity with this delightful smoothie.

Ingredient list:

- 1 cup frozen mixed berries

- 1/2 banana

- 1 cup almond milk or water

- 1 scoop of plant-based protein powder

- 1 tablespoon chia seeds

Blend until smooth. Enjoy this pop of color, flavor, and health in a glass!

The path to peak fitness is not a destination, but a journey. These shakes and smoothies offer a wonderful array of flavors while delivering a vital rush of nutrients. Experiment, twist, add, and subtract ingredients as you prefer - making these your own will enhance the journey. The key is: enjoy the process, and you'll make healthier choices more consistently.

Chapter 10. Supplements for Special Conditions: Tailoring Your Intake for Age, Sex, and Health

The beauty of nutrition lies in its adaptability. Each individual requires a distinctive set of nutrients based on several aspects – age, sex, and health condition, to name a few. This chapter encourages you to consider your specific physiological and health requirements in choosing your nutritional supplements to optimize your fitness journey.

10.1. Age and Nutritional Needs

Aging is a complex process accompanied by gradual changes in the body. As we age, our dietary needs adapt in response. Understanding this relationship between aging and nutritional needs can help effectively cater to our bodily demands and promote overall wellbeing.

10.1.1. Children and Adolescents

Children and adolescents are in their prime growth phase, with dynamic energy needs. They require ample nutrition for proper growth and development.

Essential Nutrients:

- Calcium and Vitamin D: These are vital for bone and teeth development. An excellent source of these nutrients is milk and sunlight, respectively.

- Iron: Crucial for cognitive development and immunity, iron can be obtained from sources like leafy greens and meat.

- Omega-3 Fatty Acids: These are crucial for cognitive and visual development. They can be found in flax seeds, chia seeds, and fatty fish.

- Proteins and Carbohydrates: These contribute to energy needs and support tissue growth and repair.

- Fiber: Integral for digestive health, fiber can be derived from fruits and vegetables.

- Multivitamins: To ensure comprehensive nutritional coverage, a multivitamin designed for children and adolescents could be beneficial.

Ensure to consult a healthcare provider before introducing any new supplement into your child's diet for safety and optimized dosage.

10.1.2. Adults

As we enter adulthood, the focus shifts to maintaining the state of health and preventing diseases.

Essential Nutrients:

- Calcium and Vitamin D: These are necessary to maintain bone health and prevent osteoporosis.

- B vitamins: An integral part of energy metabolism and nerve function.

- Omega-3 fatty acids: Important for cardiovascular and brain health.

- Magnesium: Necessary for muscle function and helps in relaxation.

- Fiber: Important for a healthy digestive system.

- Multivitamins: These could help cover any gaps in the diet to meet nutrient needs adequately.

Supplementing with these essential nutrients helps in maintaining good health, slowing aging, and preventing potential illnesses.

10.1.3. Seniors

Our nutritional needs continue to evolve as we approach our later years, with an increased need for certain nutrients crucial in negating age-related health complications.

Essential Nutrients:

- Vitamin B12: Necessary for brain function and energy production, but absorption often decreases with age.

- Calcium and Vitamin D: These are important for bone health to prevent osteoporosis.

- Omega-3 fatty acids: Can prevent age-related macular degeneration and support heart health.

- Fiber: Supports good digestive health.

- Probiotics: To maintain a healthy gut microbiome.

- Coenzyme Q10: Supports energy production in cells and may help slow down age-related diseases.

This general guide is a roadmap to understanding fitness in relation to age and nutritional supplements. Consult with a healthcare provider for a more personalized approach.

10.2. Gender-Specific Nutritional Needs

Men and women differ not only in anatomical and physiological attributes but also in their nutritional needs. Here's a look at how supplements can help cater to these specific needs.

10.2.1. Men

Men, particularly those engaged in high-intensity physical activities, have unique nutritional necessities.

Essential Nutrients:

- Zinc: Vital for testosterone production and immune function.
- Branched Chain Amino Acids (BCAAS): Useful for muscle recovery and growth.
- Creatine: Helps in energy production during high-intensity workouts.
- Selenium: Reduces oxidative damage and inflammation, providing muscle health benefits.

10.2.2. Women

Differences in body composition, reproductive function, and hormonal cycles induce unique nutritional requirements for women.

Essential Nutrients:

- Iron: Women, especially during childbearing age, require more iron due to menstruation.
- Calcium and Vitamin D: These are vital for bone health and can help prevent osteoporosis, more common in postmenopausal women.
- Folic Acid: Critical during pregnancy for fetal development and preventing neural tube defects.
- Omega-3 fatty acids: Supports heart health, alleviates menstrual pain, and may reduce symptoms of depression.

- Biotin: Promotes hair, skin, and nail health.

Ensure to have a discussion with your healthcare provider to better understand your individual nutritional needs.

10.3. Tailoring Supplements for Specific Health Conditions

Nutrition can play an instrumental role in managing and improving various health conditions. Here are some health-specific considerations.

10.3.1. Heart Health

- Omega-3 fatty acids: Reduces inflammation and risks of developing heart diseases.

- Coenzyme Q10: Might help improve symptoms of congestive heart failure.

- Folic Acid, B6, and B12 vitamins: Can potentially lower the risk of heart disease.

- Magnesium: May help in maintaining a normal heart rhythm.

10.3.2. Bone and Joint Health

- Calcium and Vitamin D: Essential for bone health.

- Glucosamine and Chondroitin: Can support joint health and slow degradation.

- Vitamin K: Plays a key role in helping the body absorb calcium.

When dealing with specific health conditions, always consult your healthcare provider before introducing supplements. It is crucial to remember that while supplements can support health, they should not replace traditional therapies unless directed by your healthcare provider.

In summary, tailoring your supplement intake can be a game-changer in your fitness journey. Empowered with accurate knowledge of supplements, you can truly align your nutrition with your unique body needs. It's time to make informed choices and ascend on your path to optimum health and fitness.

Chapter 11. Setting and Tracking Your Fitness Goals: A Roadmap to Success with Flex Nutrition

A goal is not merely a pit stop in the grand journey of life. It is a collaboratively planned pursuit that requires determination, patience, and a touch of adventure-driven enthusiasm for enduring the entire path. As you embark on your fitness journey, there are essential guidelines to follow, and at the heart of it is Flex Nutrition. Tailoring the science of nutrition to your individual needs and aspirations, we offer a powerful tool at your disposal.

11.1. Necessity of Goal Setting

The establishment of a goal is the first step towards a successful fitness journey. Common fitness goals might include weight loss, gaining muscle, improving cardiovascular health or increasing strength. Whatever it may be, it's significant because it provides direction to your efforts. It serves as the guiding star along your journey; whenever you feel lost, you can rely on your goal to redirect your efforts.

It's important to remember that a goal is not a destination, but a journey in itself. It's a promise to yourself, a commitment to improve, to grow, and to be better than you were before. It's a contract of self-improvement that you sign with yourself, promising to persevere and pull through.

11.2. Crafting Your Fitness Goals

Here, the key is striking the balance between aspiration and realistic evaluation. You need to have a vision that motivates and inspires you, but at the same time, it needs to be grounded in reality.

While framing your goal, follow the S.M.A.R.T principle - make it Specific, Measurable, Achievable, Relevant, and Time-bound. It's not enough to have a goal of "getting fit"; you need to specify what fitness means to you. Is it achieving a certain weight, lifting a certain amount of weight, or running a specific distance? "Measurable" allows for the tracking of progress and gives a clear picture of where you stand. "Achievable" refers to setting goals within your capabilities. "Relevant" ensures the goal aligns with your lifestyle, values and broader objectives. "Time-bound" adds a sense of urgency and prompts you to take action.

For instance, a well-framed goal might be "losing 10 pounds in six months through strength training and nutritional changes". The goal is detailed and provides a clear pathway.

11.3. Empowering Through Flex Nutrition

Flex Nutrition comes into play by providing the necessary nutritional support for your fitness goals. A well-managed diet can significantly enhance your performance, recovery, and overall progress.

Flex Nutrition's products are designed to meet different nutritional demands - from weight loss to muscle gain and everything in between. Protein powders, multivitamin tablets, pre-workout supplements - you name it, Flex Nutrition has it for you.

To meet the nutritional demands of a goal like "losing 10 pounds in six months", calorie intake and expenditure play a vital role. Flex

Nutrition's guidance helps you understand the proper balance between them, avoiding excessive calorie restriction and promoting an active lifestyle.

11.4. Tracking Your Goals with Flex Nutrition

Tracking your progress is a fundamental part of this journey; it ignites enthusiasm by revealing improvements, no matter how small. The nuances of physiological variations make it crucial to subject your body to regular check-ups.

Here's a systematic structure to follow:

1. Establish Baseline Measurements: Start with recording all the related metrics - weight, body composition, body measurements, strength levels, endurance levels, etc., and periodic re-evaluations.

2. Keep a Training Log: Maintain a detailed account of your workout regime, this helps identify if changes are needed based on performance progress.

3. Monitor Your Nutrition: Alongside training, monitoring your diet composition is crucial. Keep track of protein, fat, and carbohydrate intake and align it with your workout.

4. Scheduled Macros and Micros: On the lines of Flex Nutrition, you need to have a well-scheduled intake of your macronutrients (proteins, fats, and carbs) and micronutrients (essential vitamins and minerals).

5. Compare Progress with Goal: Regularly compare your current standing with the end goal. If there are discrepancies, re-work your strategies.

Launching an expedition towards your fitness goals requires

courage, and maintaining the trajectory mandates steadfast discipline. While the journey may seem overwhelming, the potential rewards are invaluable. You gain not just physical fitness, but a new relationship with self-discipline, willpower, and perseverance.

In the end, the golden rule for everyone, despite the specific goals, is to listen to your body. Every body is unique and responds differently to various diets, exercises, and supplements. Flex Nutrition understands this and emphasizes the benefits of personalized fitness solutions.

Find what works for you, set your goals, and push your boundaries because a fitter version of yourself is awaiting you, just a few steps away. Let Flex Nutrition and this guide be your trusted companions in this exciting journey and soon, you'll find that the journey itself is the reward.